Methylene Blue Unveiled

A Comprehensive Guide to its Chemistry, Health Benefits, and Applications

Dr. Smith Harvey

Table of Contents

Introduction

Historical Overview and Background on Methylene Blue

Methylene blue is a synthetic dye that has been used for over 100 years across a variety of applications. The history of methylene blue provides insights into its versatility as a stain, antiseptic, and therapeutic agent.

Methylene blue was first synthesized in 1876 by German chemist Heinrich Caro. He was working on developing new textile dyes and created methylene blue as a byproduct. Its vibrant blue color and staining abilities quickly made it popular as a biological stain. By the 1880s, methylene blue was being widely used to stain bacteria and tissues for microscopic study. Early pioneers of microbiology and histology relied on methylene blue as an essential dye for visualizing cells and microorganisms.

In the 1890s, methylene blue found an additional crucial application - as an antiseptic and antimalarial agent. Doctors and pharmacists began using dilute methylene blue solutions for disinfecting skin and sterilizing surgical instruments. At around the same time, researchers discovered that methylene blue could kill the malaria parasite Plasmodium at certain concentrations. This made it useful as a treatment for malaria, which was a widespread and deadly disease at the time. Though replaced by alternative methods in malaria treatment, Methylene Blue persisted in the medical field.

In the early twentieth century, methylene blue's applications further expanded due to its redox capabilities. Scientists found it could act as an electron transfer agent and mild mitochondrial inhibitor inside cells. These properties suggested methylene blue might have therapeutic effects for conditions related to cellular respiration and oxidative stress. By the 1930s-40s, physicians occasionally gave intravenous methylene blue to patients suffering from conditions like cyanide poisoning to attempt respiratory stimulation.

Most recently, methylene blue has re-emerged as a topic of research for several neurological diseases. Recent evidence indicates methylene blue is a tau aggregation inhibitor, meaning it can prevent pathological tau proteins from aggregating in the brain. Since the 2000s, numerous clinical trials have been conducted examining methylene blue's effects on tauopathic diseases such as Alzheimer's disease and frontotemporal dementia. Though outcomes have been mixed so far, its long history paints methylene blue as a versatile small molecule with broad therapeutic potential.

Over its 150-year history, methylene blue has been an invaluable stain, antiseptic tool, antimalarial therapy, mitochondrial modulator and oxidant scavenger. Now both its known bioactivities and new ones continue to be investigated, opening more possibilities for this historically useful dye. From textile factories to operating rooms to pharmacology labs, researchers continue discovering methylene blue's varied applications.

CHAPTER 1

The Chemistry of Methylene Blue

As we embark on this exploration, we would look into the intricate molecular world that defines the essence of Methylene Blue. Within this chapter, we will dissect its chemical composition through three key lenses – 1.1 Molecular Structure, unveiling the tricyclic aromatic system and the pivotal nitrogen atom orchestrating electron transfer; 1.2 General Properties, shedding light on its solubility and stability, crucial aspects shaping its utility; and 1.3 Trade Names, recognizing the compound beyond its chemical formula.

Molecular Structure

Methylene blue, beyond its captivating blue hue, boasts a fascinating molecular structure that underpins its diverse properties and applications. This intricate dance of atoms and bonds forms the bedrock of its chemical identity.

At a fundamental level, methylene blue is a heterocyclic aromatic chemical compound with the chemical formula $C_{16}H_{18}N_3SCl$. Breaking down this formula reveals key elements that contribute to its distinctive properties. Composed of carbon (C), hydrogen (H), nitrogen (N), sulfur (S), and chlorine (Cl) atoms, the molecular arrangement of methylene blue is a captivating interplay of these elements.

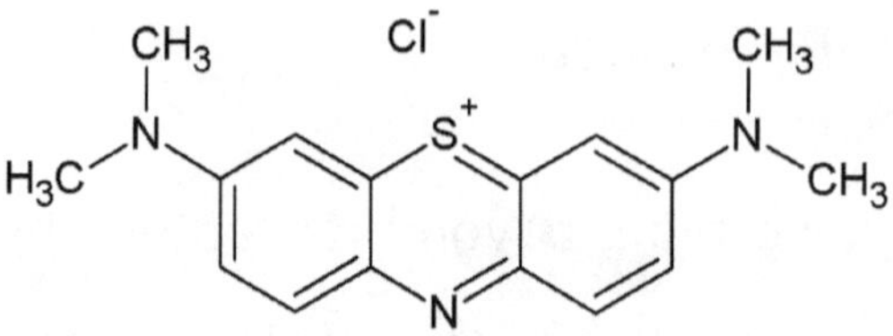

The aromaticity of methylene blue arises from its heterocyclic nature, featuring a planar aromatic ring system. The conjugation of double bonds within this system contributes to its characteristic blue color and enhances its stability. The resonance effect in the aromatic ring structure creates a delocalized electron cloud, reinforcing the compound's overall stability.

The central core of methylene blue consists of a thiazine ring, which comprises four nitrogen and two carbon atoms. This thiazine ring forms the backbone of the compound, providing a stable platform for various functional groups and interactions. The arrangement of these atoms not only imparts structural integrity but also influences the compound's reactivity.

Adjacent to the thiazine ring is a phenothiazine moiety, characterized by its fused aromatic rings. This structural motif significantly contributes to methylene blue's absorption and emission properties. The phenothiazine unit is essential for its role as a redox-active compound, making methylene blue a valuable electron transfer mediator in biological and chemical processes.

Introducing the sulfur atom within the thiazine ring adds a distinctive element to methylene blue's chemical makeup. The sulfur atom serves as a key player in redox reactions, facilitating electron transfer and contributing to the compound's ability to act as an electron carrier in various biological systems.

The chlorine atom in the molecular formula is a halogen element that plays a crucial role in fine-tuning the chemical and physical properties of methylene blue. This halogen contributes to the compound's solubility, stability, and reactivity, influencing its behavior in different environments.

Understanding the molecular structure of methylene blue is paramount for unlocking its myriad applications. In medicine, it serves as a vital staining agent for histological studies, aiding in the visualization of cellular structures. In the field of chemistry, its redox properties find utility in electron transfer reactions and analytical techniques.

General Properties

Methylene Blue (MB), a versatile dye and pharmaceutical agent, boasts a rich array of general properties that underscore its extensive applications. Known for its distinctive blue hue, MB is a heterocyclic aromatic compound characterized by a planar aromatic ring system. This structural feature, marked by the conjugation of double bonds, contributes to the compound's remarkable stability, a trait that extends to its water solubility—critical for its multifaceted use.

Central to MB's appeal is its notable redox activity. Methylene blue possesses a unique ability to switch between its oxidized (blue) and reduced (colorless) forms. The compound readily engages in reversible reduction-oxidation reactions, positioning it as an invaluable electron carrier in both biological and chemical realms. This redox capability has propelled MB into various applications, ranging from its traditional role in histological staining to serving as a redox indicator in analytical chemistry. Notably, this property also holds significant therapeutic potential, as its reduced form exhibits promising biological activities currently under investigation.

The absorption and emission properties of MB, attributed to its phenothiazine moiety, elevate its significance in biomedical applications. The compound's involvement in photodynamic therapy, wherein its absorption of light leads to the generation of reactive oxygen species for therapeutic purposes, underscores its pivotal role in medical treatments. Additionally, MB's application as a contrast agent in medical imaging relies on these optical properties.

The permeability of MB through biological membranes enhances its utility in cellular studies, allowing researchers to investigate intracellular processes. This characteristic, combined with its photodynamic properties, positions MB as a tool for targeted interventions at the cellular level.

Thermal Stability: Methylene blue possesses a relatively high melting point, typically ranging from 100-110°C. This thermal stability ensures its structural integrity during various applications, such as in dyeing textiles or as a component in analytical chemistry experiments. Furthermore, its resistance to thermal degradation contributes to its extended shelf life, making it a reliable tool for scientific endeavors.

Beyond its biological applications, MB finds utility in various industrial processes, showcasing its adaptability across scientific and industrial domains. Its use as a redox mediator extends to applications in batteries and electrochemical systems, highlighting its impact in energy-related fields.

CHAPTER 2

Methylene Blue As A Dye

Of all the many uses of methylene blue over the past 130 years, its original and most long-standing function has been as a blue dye for staining fabrics and fibers across a range of industries. The vivid and stable coloration produced by methylene blue has made it an essential component for applications as varied as dyeing cotton in textile manufacturing to selectively staining paper and fibers in forensic investigations.

The unique chemical attributes of methylene blue that make it amendable as a versatile dye are its highly conjugated aromatic structure and electrophilic properties. These enable methylene blue to bind securely and robustly to materials containing electron-rich functional groups such as phenols, anilines, and aromatic amines. As such, methylene blue is defined as a basic dye with a strong attraction toward cellulosic plant fibers, silk, nylon, and other substances rich in aromatic moieties or negatively-charged sites. The strength and longevity of such binding to fabric and fiber substrates give finished materials colored by methylene blue excellent wash-fastness ratings.

One of the earliest and most common applications of the dye has been in dyeing cotton, wool, and silk fabrics with a range of rich blues. The tint may range from pale shade to a nearly black midnight blue depending on factors such as dye concentration, fabric composition, and mordant usage. In textile dyeing, methylene blue is typically applied using immersion or continuous dyeing methods with other auxiliary chemicals and temperature control to facilitate bonding to fibers. The exceptional penetration into dense and complex fabrics made methylene blue invaluable for uniform coloration of textiles prior to the advent of many synthetic fiber dyes.

Beyond fabric dyeing, methylene blue also serves highly specialized niches in directly dyeing or enhancing the finishing of paper products. Paper and boards containing lignin or unbleached pulp components have affinity for methylene blue, allowing selective shading. Artists, decorators, and forensic examiners apply aqueous or alcohol solutions containing very dilute methylene blue when selective staining of paper fibers, patterns, or fingerprints is needed for aesthetic and investigative purposes. Such vanishingly small quantities of dye minimize risks for paper degradation over time.

The capacity to produce intense, lasting shades on both natural and synthetic materials at minute concentrations has thus ensured methylene blue a enduring central role as a versatile and economical tinting agent now in its second century of dyestuff applications. Ongoing uses in emerging areas like photosensitized fabrics and microencapsulated dyes suggest even broader horizons ahead for this deeply-hued dye.

Use in Textile Dyeing

As one of the earliest synthetic dyes, methylene blue rapidly became indispensable in the textile industry for dyeing cotton, linen, rayon, wool, and silk. The dye stuff works well across a broad range of fibers at nearly neutral pH using mordants like tannin or metal salts to fix color. Even today, methylene blue remains a widely used bargain dye for producing shades of blue economically from light sky tones to dark navy hues across all manner of fabrics. However, being a basic dye, methylene blue requires special cationic fixatives when used to color fabrics containing acetyl groups like polyesters or acid-modified nylons, limiting utility for synthetic blends.

Photographic Uses

Early in photography's history, very dilute solutions of methylene blue were employed as a blue tinting agent for sepia images and prints lacking cool hues. Later, methylene blue found an important role in cyanotype photographic printing which produces vivid white-on-blue pictures. The printing process coats paper with ferric salts, then exposes coated paper to UV light which selectively converts methylene blue in masked areas from nearly colorless leuco form to intensely blue oxidized pigment. Once popular with engineers requiring durable blueprints, modern creative uses of cyanotype's stark contrast include decorative photographic art, textile dying, and botanical imprinting kits using the versatile, long-lived print chemistry enabled by methylene blue's photoswitching redox magic.

Biological Staining Applications

One of the earliest and still most common uses for aqueous or alcohol-based methylene blue solutions is selective staining of tissue samples on microscope slides and in laboratory cell preparations. Often used as a contrasting counterstain to eosin or safranin, methylene blue binds to negatively charged cell components like DNA/RNA, rendering nuclei and mitochondria vivid blue against pink backdrops under magnification. The same ionic attraction allows methylene blue to subtly highlight paper fibers and fingerprints by optical microscopy methods valuable in forensic work. So indispensable for cellular structures, living bacteria, and protein localizations, microbiology and clinical labs worldwide depend daily on methylene blue's staining prowess—a testament to the dye's bioaffinity cemented now for multiple centuries.

CHAPTER 3

Comparisons with Alternative Dyes and Stains

As a dye and biological stain, methylene blue exhibits a number of distinct advantages over other options in terms of safety, versatility, and imaging outcome quality. However, no single dye molecule is perfectly suited to all possible staining situations or exploration goals encountered in industrial, research, medical, or scientific realms. Thus, alternative dyes offer their own benefits in select scenarios depending on the substrate material, the type of optical differentiation desired, and even budget constraints. Often, employing multiple compatible dyes together leads to superior, synergistic stains than a single agent alone might achieve.

Advantages Over Other Histological Stains

Methylene blue has distinguished itself as a dye especially amenable to and invaluable for biological imaging applications spanning histology, hematology, microbiology, and cytology. For well over a century, it has served as a prototype for an industry-standard histological stain offering numerous benefits for researchers and clinicians:

Safety and Appropriate Toxicity Profile - At appropriate dilute concentrations for staining, methylene blue demonstrates remarkably low toxicity to healthy mammalian cells and tissues while potently disrupting pathogens and diseased cells through oxidative damage. This allows methylene blue to selectively visualize desired bio-targets without harming specimens.

Rapid Staining - Unlike some stains requiring prolonged development or lengthy de-staining, methylene blue often colors specimens in minutes with the depth of shade indicating degree of uptake by cells and structures of interest. This enables rapid staining assessment.

Color Intensity and Photostability - The tinctorial power of methylene blue stems from its brilliant hue and resistance to fading even under intense or prolonged light irradiation. This benefits specimen imaging quality and archival storage.

Enhanced Contrast - Methylene blue produces an intense blue color that contrasts strongly against eosin (pink) and provides negative image staining that complements brown pigments like DAB. This amplifies specimen feature differentiation.

Cost Effectiveness - As one of the earliest synthetic dyes, methylene blue became affordable to produce at industrial scales. This makes it a budget-friendly choice compatible with high through-put testing.

Adaptability - Methylene blue readily stains a wide range of tissues, cell types, and bacteria across plant, animal, and fungal samples using routine protocols. Ease of use lowers training barriers.

Situations Where Other Dyes Excel

That said, methylene blue does suffer some comparative limitations against emerging contemporary alternatives that may excel in specific situations:

Fluorescent Dyes - For advanced high-resolution microscopy techniques like confocal scanning, fluorescent markers like DAPI offer sharper signaling specificity and multiplex advantages over conventional dyes.

Automated Analysis - Some colorimetric reagents amenable to spectrophotometric quantification in microplate assays provide more objective analytical power along with high-throughput capacities.

Ultrafine Discrimination - Related thiazine dyes better differentiate intricate neuroanatomical, myelin, and neuralgia features crucial in neural pathology investigations.

Non-Destructive Testing - Dyes permitting visualization in biofilms, seed coats, and live-tissue culture without deleterious effects uniquely enable non-invasive study of undamaged structures.

Synthetic Affinity - Select basic and disperse dyes form tenacious covalent bonds with synthetics like nylon, PVC, acrylic, and polyester that surpass methylene blue's reliance on ionic interactions with material substrates.

Complementary Mixed Staining

While no single dye solution ideally satisfies every possible research or clinical situation, combining methylene blue with compatible contrasting dyes creates complementary staining outcomes unattainable through solitary agents. Taking advantage of the distinct binding preferences and spectral properties of individual dyes expands the palette for differentiated visualization.

Common examples of synergistic co-staining leveraging methylene blue's capabilities alongside other dye stuffs include:

- Methylene blue + Eosin - Highlights cytoplasmic and intracellular features against pink connective tissue backdrops

- Methylene blue + Safranin - Detects fungal organism morphology and associated tissue inflammation

- Methylene blue + Crystal violet - Mixed to create Wright's stain solution for blood smears and bone marrow samples

- Methylene blue + Rhodamine B - Fluorescent amplified staining for cancerous tissue margins

- Methylene blue + Congo Red - Identifies aberrant protein aggregation typical in amyloids

- Methylene blue + Celestine blue - Binds age pigment lipofuscin accumulation over time

- Methylene blue + Neutral red - Visualizes live vs dead cell populations in culture

The unique chemical attributes of methylene blue will continue catalyzing ongoing dye chemistry innovations well into the future. But even as new stains emerge, methylene blue endures as a trusted, flexible, and economical dye synergist ready to combine forces with complementary colorants across unforeseeable staining frontiers.

CHAPTER 4

Medical Uses

Early Medical Applications

The early medical applications of Methylene Blue reveal a dynamic history of experimentation and adaptation, showcasing the compound's versatility and adaptability in the realm of healthcare. Originating as a laboratory dye, Methylene Blue quickly transcended its initial purpose, finding its way into the hands of pioneering medical practitioners in the late 19th century.

One of the earliest medical applications of Methylene Blue was in the realm of infectious diseases. In 1891, it earned its place in medical history as one of the first chemotherapeutic agents tested in humans. During this era, the compound underwent trials for the treatment of malaria, a prevalent and challenging infectious disease. While Methylene Blue eventually yielded to alternative methods for malaria treatment, the early trials laid the foundation for its exploration in various medical avenues.

The compound's staining properties, initially designed for microbes in the laboratory, found unexpected utility in medical diagnostics. Pathologists began utilizing Methylene Blue as a stain in histopathology, enhancing the visualization of cellular structures and aiding in the identification of various tissues and pathogens under the microscope. This application not only improved diagnostic accuracy but also contributed to the advancement of medical knowledge.

Furthermore, Methylene Blue's unique chemical properties led to its use in addressing cyanide poisoning. The compound acts as a chemical reducer, aiding in the conversion of toxic cyanide into less harmful substances within the body. This property became particularly relevant in emergency situations where rapid intervention was crucial.

As medical knowledge expanded, so did the understanding of Methylene Blue's potential applications. The compound found utility in treating conditions such as septic shock, where its ability to improve cellular oxygen utilization became a valuable asset. The early medical applications of Methylene Blue laid the groundwork for its evolving role in critical care and emergency medicine.

The compound's adaptability didn't stop there; it continued to be explored in diverse medical contexts, including its potential neuroprotective effects in conditions such as Alzheimer's disease. These early applications paved the way for ongoing research and highlighted the compound's multifaceted nature in addressing a spectrum of medical challenges.

FDA Approval for Methemoglobinemia

The FDA approval for Methylene Blue in the treatment of methemoglobinemia marks a significant milestone in the compound's medical journey. Methemoglobinemia is a rare blood disorder where an abnormal amount of methemoglobin, a form of hemoglobin, is present. This condition impairs the blood's ability to release oxygen to tissues, leading to symptoms such as fatigue, cyanosis, and shortness of breath.

Methylene Blue, initially developed as a laboratory dye, found its therapeutic niche in addressing methemoglobinemia. The compound acts as a reducing agent, aiding in the conversion of methemoglobin back to functional hemoglobin, which can effectively transport oxygen. This unique property became the basis for seeking regulatory approval.

In 2011, the U.S. Food and Drug Administration (FDA) officially approved

Methylene Blue for the treatment of methemoglobinemia. This endorsement underscored the compound's safety, efficacy, and the crucial role it plays in managing this rare blood disorder.

The approval was grounded in comprehensive clinical trials that demonstrated Methylene Blue's effectiveness in rapidly reversing methemoglobinemia-induced hypoxia. The intravenous administration of Methylene Blue emerged as a reliable and expedient intervention, particularly in cases where traditional treatments, such as oxygen therapy, were insufficient.

Beyond its primary use, the FDA approval also paved the way for exploring Methylene

Blue's potential applications in other medical contexts. Researchers and clinicians began to investigate its utility in various conditions, including septic shock and vasoplegic syndrome, further expanding its therapeutic repertoire.

The FDA's imprimatur solidified Methylene Blue's status as a medically valuable agent, extending its reach beyond the laboratory setting into the realm of critical medical interventions. The endorsement emphasized the compound's safety profile when administered under controlled conditions, providing healthcare professionals with a reliable tool in managing a challenging hematological condition.

CHAPTER 5
Potential Health Benefits of Methylene Blue

Methylene blue, a vibrant molecule with a long history, has garnered attention for its potential health benefits. However, it's crucial to approach this topic with caution, acknowledging the absence of conclusive evidence and the need for further research.

Several areas demonstrate promising preliminary findings, but require extensive clinical trials for confirmation. These include:

- **Neurological Disorders**: Studies suggest potential in addressing

Alzheimer's and Parkinson's, but these remain exploratory and inconclusive.

- **Mood Disorders**: Early investigations hint at possible improvements in depression and anxiety symptoms, but long-term safety and efficacy remain unknown.

- **Infectious Diseases**: Methylene blue's antimicrobial properties might combat certain infections, but its effectiveness and potential drug interactions require thorough evaluation.

It's essential to emphasize that currently, methylene blue is not approved for most of these potential uses. Additionally, self-administration is strongly discouraged due to potential risks and side effects.

Research on methylene blue's health benefits is ongoing, and future studies might uncover valuable applications. However, consulting a healthcare professional is paramount before considering its use for any health concern. They can provide qualified advice based on current evidence and your individual needs.

Cognitive Function

Age-related cognitive decline and neurodegenerative diseases like Alzheimer's and Parkinson's are characterized by the progressive loss of neurons. As a neuroprotective agent that easily crosses the blood-brain barrier, methylene blue shows promise for enhancing and preserving cognitive abilities.

Through its action on critical cellular pathways, methylene blue demonstrates several properties that support healthy brain cell function. As a mitochondrial enhancer, methylene blue boosts energy production which is essential for fueling neurotransmission, plasticity mechanisms, and repair processes in the brain. It also functions as an antioxidant and anti-inflammatory molecule that defends neurons from oxidative stress and neuroinflammation – common drivers of neurodegeneration. Furthermore, methylene blue is a potent stimulator of cellular degradative pathways like autophagy. Upkeeping efficient protein and organelle turnover is vital for neurons overloaded with misfolded proteins in aging. By bolstering mitochondria, reducing inflammation, and stimulating waste clearance, methylene blue creates favorable cellular conditions for neurons to thrive.

In preclinical studies of Alzheimer's, Parkinson's, and stroke models, methylene blue improved memory, learning, sensory perception, and motor function. It stimulated neuron growth and communication while reducing brain plaque levels and oxidative damage. In elderly non-demented adults, short-term methylene blue administration heightened memory, executive function, and processing speed. Ongoing research examines its long-term benefits.

While small early trials reported faster processing speed and attention switching, additional large clinical trials are required to confirm effects on normal age-related cognitive decline and neurodegenerative trajectories. For its modulation of major pathways implicated in neurodegeneration, methylene blue remains a promising therapeutic candidate to boost and protcct cognition throughout the aging process.

Alzheimer's Disease

Alzheimer's disease (AD) is characterized by progressive neuronal damage and loss due to the accumulation of tau protein tangles and amyloid beta plaques in the brain. As a small molecule that can cross the blood-brain barrier, methylene blue is uniquely poised to impact disease progression in AD.

Methylene blue has demonstrated several beneficial mechanisms of action for alleviating underlying causes of AD pathology. First, methylene blue acts as a tau protein aggregator inhibitor by preventing the abnormal phosphorylation and aggregation of tau proteins into neurofibrillary tangles. By inhibiting tau tangles, methylene blue can slow neuronal dysfunction and death. Second, methylene blue enhances mitochondrial function and cellular metabolism which is often impaired early in disease. Boosting mitochondrial efficiency increases available energy for neuron functioning. Finally, methylene blue functions as a potent antioxidant and anti-inflammatory agent which reduces oxidative damage and neuroinflammation. Excess inflammation accelerates neuronal injury.

Multiple preclinical studies in animal models of AD-like pathology found that methylene blue improved memory deficits, reduced tauopathy, decreased oxidant damage and amyloid beta levels, increased cerebral blood flow and mitochondrial activity, and protected neuron health and lifespan.

Early clinical trials in humans found some preliminary evidence that short-term methylene blue treatment potentially improves cognitive scores in people with AD, though results remain mixed on efficacy so far. Future large-scale trials are underway to provide more thorough testing. With its multimodal mechanisms to address contributors to AD progression and neuron death, methylene blue offers promise as a therapeutic intervention.

Septic Shock

Sepsis occurs when an infection triggers an overwhelming inflammatory response, leading to life-threatening organ dysfunction. In septic shock, blood pressure severely drops, hindering oxygen delivery to the body's vital organs. With mortality rates upwards of 40%, effective interventions for septic shock are desperately needed.

As a potent anti-inflammatory and oxidant scavenger, methylene blue shows promise for mitigating septic shock severity and damage. During septic shock, widespread inflammation triggers nitric oxide overproduction. Excess nitric oxide impairs vascular tone regulation, causing drastic blood pressure decreases. By inhibiting nitric oxide production, methylene blue can attenuate hypotension episodes in septic shock. Additionally, unrestrained inflammation generates free radicals that destroy proteins, DNA, and lipids essential for normal cell functioning. As an antioxidant, methylene blue neutralizes these cell-damaging free radicals. Oxidative damage to mitochondria is especially deleterious, limiting energy availability in cells already struggling from poor perfusion. By preserving mitochondrial function, methylene blue aids in meeting cells' high energy demands during sepsis.

Beyond its anti-inflammatory and antioxidant properties, methylene blue helps maintain critical oxygen delivery to tissues. In red blood cells, methylene blue accepts electrons from metabolic coenzymes and delivers them to molecular oxygen - transforming it into readily available oxygen. This oxygenating capability helps sustain oxygen supply to vital organs that would otherwise suffer from septic shock's drastic drop in blood pressure.

Several clinical studies found infusion of methylene blue increased blood pressure, reduced vasopressor needs, and improved kidney and liver function in septic shock patients. More research is underway, but methylene blue's multimodal protection shows early promise against septic shock and its life-threatening consequences. By combating hypotension, oxidative damage, and hypoxia, methylene blue has emerging potential to improve outcomes for this deadly manifestation of sepsis.

Other Health Conditions

Beyond its applications in Alzheimer's disease and sepsis, emerging research highlights the versatile therapeutic potential of methylene blue across an array of disease states.

Methylene blue's antioxidant and electron-transport properties are under investigation for uses in cardiovascular disease for improving heart function post-injury and protecting heart tissue during cardiac surgery requiring an abrupt halt in blood flow. Additionally, methylene blue shows early promise as an oral supplement for enhancing muscular endurance during exercise by making oxygen utilization more efficient.

Within cancer research, methylene blue is re-emerging for its selective toxicity toward cancer cells over healthy cells. As an alternative redox modulating therapy, methylene blue increased tumor response to radiation in clinical studies by heightening oxidative stress specifically in cancer cells. Combining methylene blue with existing treatments may allow lower therapeutic doses and mitigate side effects.

In psychiatry, methylene blue's impact on modulating brain monoamine oxidase enzymes led to trials for depression which found faster remission for methylene blue versus placebo when enhancing standard antidepressants. Case reports note benefits also for stabilizing mood disorders like bipolar disease.

With antimicrobial actions coupled to its oxidant properties, topical or oral methylene blue improves wound healing for burns, abrasions, and ulcers by reducing microbial load and infection risk. This supports its use for treating stubborn gastrointestinal infections caused by bacteria or parasites without excess antibiotics.

While research continues elucidating mechanisms, the unique biochemistry of methylene blue unlocks opportunities across specialties, including cardiology, exercise physiology, oncology, psychiatry, and infectious disease. Its versatile therapeutic potential parlays a long history of chemical serendipity into clinical promise.

CHAPTER 6

Side Effects and Risks

Methylene blue, with its diverse applications and promising research, carries inherent side effects and potential risks that demand careful consideration. While exploring its potential benefits, responsible awareness of these limitations is crucial.

Gastrointestinal Side Effects of Methylene Blue: Understanding the Gut Impact

Though generally well-tolerated, some individuals may experience mild gastrointestinal discomfort as a result of Methylene Blue administration. While understanding these effects is crucial before considering this compound for any medical use, it's essential to emphasize that methylene blue is not currently approved for most of these potential uses and self-administration is strictly discouraged due to safety concerns.

Common GI Side Effects:

- **Nausea and Vomiting**: These are the most frequent GI complaints associated with methylene blue, occurring in up to 20% of patients. The mechanisms behind these effects are not fully understood, but they might involve stimulation of the vagus nerve or direct irritation of the gut lining.
- **Abdominal Pain and Discomfort**: Cramping, bloating, and general abdominal discomfort are also

reported by some individuals, potentially due to altered gut motility or inflammation.

- **Diarrhea**: Loose stools or increased bowel frequency can occur, primarily due to changes in fluid and electrolyte balance within the intestines.

These effects are typically transient and tend to subside once the compound is metabolized within the body.

Severity and Contributing Factors:

The severity and occurrence of GI side effects vary widely across individuals. Factors influencing their likelihood include:

- **Dosage**: Higher doses tend to increase the risk and intensity of GI effects.

- **Route of Administration**: Oral administration generally exhibits the highest incidence of GI side effects compared to other routes like injection or topical application.

- **Individual Sensitivity**: Some individuals have a higher susceptibility to gastrointestinal irritation from medications, including methylene blue.

- **Concurrent Medications**: Interactions with other medications, particularly those affecting gut motility or digestion, can exacerbate GI side effects.

Management and Mitigation:

While research on mitigating GI side effects of methylene blue is ongoing, some potential strategies might offer relief:

- **Lowering the Dose**: Reducing the dosage can significantly decrease the risk and severity of GI effects.
- **Splitting Doses**: Administering the medication in smaller, divided doses throughout the day may improve tolerance.
- **Taking with Food**: Consuming food alongside methylene blue might reduce irritation to the stomach lining.
- **Anti-Nausea Medications**: In some cases, healthcare professionals might prescribe anti-nausea medication to manage symptoms.

Neurological Side Effects

One notable neurological side effect is the development of serotonin syndrome. Methylene Blue has the potential to inhibit the enzyme monoamine oxidase (MAO), leading to an increase in serotonin levels. In conjunction with other serotonergic medications, this elevation may contribute to serotonin syndrome, a condition characterized by symptoms such as agitation, confusion, rapid heartbeat, and in severe cases, hyperthermia. This risk underscores the importance of cautious use, particularly when Methylene Blue is administered concomitantly with other medications affecting serotonin levels.

Common Neurological Side Effects:

- **Headache and Dizziness**: These are the most frequent neurological complaints, occurring in up to 15% of individuals. Increased blood pressure or direct effects on the nervous system might contribute to these symptoms.

- **Confusion and Anxiety**: In rare instances, altered mental clarity, restlessness, and even hallucinations can occur, potentially due to interactions with brain chemistry or imbalances in neurotransmitters. These effects are typically dose-dependent and reversible upon discontinuation of Methylene Blue.

- **Insomnia and Sleep Disturbances**: Difficulty falling asleep or maintaining sleep can arise from nervous system stimulation or changes in brain activity.

Understanding Individual Risks:

Factors influencing the likelihood and severity of neurological side effects include:

- **Dosage**: Higher doses increase the risk and intensity of effects.
- **Underlying Conditions**: Pre-existing neurological issues or sensitivity to specific medications can make individuals more susceptible.
- **Drug Interactions**: Concomitant medications can interact with methylene blue, potentially amplifying neurological side effects.

Management and Minimizing Risks:

While research on mitigating neurological side effects is ongoing, some potential approaches might offer relief:

- **Dose Reduction**: Lowering the dose often reduces the risk and severity of neurological effects.
- **Monitoring**: Close monitoring of symptoms by a healthcare professional is crucial.
- **Discontinuation**: If severe or persistent neurological side effects occur, stopping the medication is essential.

Understanding and monitoring neurological side effects are paramount during the administration of Methylene Blue, especially in contexts where the compound is used for conditions beyond its FDA-approved indications, such as in experimental or investigational therapies.

Healthcare providers exercise prudence in assessing patient medical histories and potential drug interactions to minimize the risk of neurological side effects. Close monitoring for signs of serotonin syndrome and other neurological manifestations is essential, particularly in patients with pre-existing neurological conditions or those on medications that could potentiate such effects.

Urinary Side Effects

Methylene blue, while demonstrating potential in various research areas, including urinary tract infections, comes with potential side effects impacting the very system it targets.

Spectrum of Urinary Concerns:

Urinary side effects associated with methylene blue, though generally transient, can cause discomfort and require awareness:

- **Discoloration**: The most frequent effect, turning urine bright blue or green due to the compound's inherent color, is harmless and resolves upon discontinuation.
- **Urinary Tract Irritation**: Burning, stinging, or discomfort during urination might occur, potentially arising from mild inflammation of the bladder or urinary tract lining.

- **Frequency and Urgency**: Increased urination and a persistent urge to void can manifest, possibly linked to direct bladder stimulation or changes in fluid balance.

Understanding Individual Vulnerability:

The likelihood and severity of these side effects depend on various factors:

- **Dosage**: Higher doses increase the risk and intensity of urinary effects.
- **Route of Administration**: Oral administration generally exhibits the highest incidence of urinary side effects compared to other routes like injection.
- **Underlying Conditions**: Individuals with pre-existing urinary tract issues

or sensitivities might be more susceptible.

- **Drug Interactions**: Concomitant medications can interact with methylene blue, potentially amplifying urinary side effects.

Strategies for Mitigation:

While research on managing urinary side effects of methylene blue remains ongoing, some potential approaches might offer relief:

- **Dose Reduction**: Lowering the dose often reduces the risk and intensity of urinary effects.
- **Hydration**: Increased fluid intake helps dilute the concentration of methylene blue in the urine, potentially minimizing irritation.

- **Symptomatic Relief**: If discomfort persists, over-the-counter pain relievers or medications prescribed by a healthcare professional might offer relief.

Side Effects Pertaining to the Skin

Methylene blue, while possessing potential in various research areas, carries potential side effects impacting the very system it interacts with - the skin. Understanding these risks and advocating for responsible exploration are crucial before considering this molecule for any health concern.

Spectrum of Skin Concerns:

Skin side effects associated with methylene blue vary in severity and can range from mild discoloration to more serious reactions:

- **Discoloration**: The most frequent effect, turning skin a blue-green hue due to the compound's inherent color, is usually temporary and resolves upon discontinuation.
- **Contact Dermatitis**: Itching, redness, and burning at the application site can occur, potentially indicating an allergic reaction or irritation.
- **Photosensitivity**: Increased skin sensitivity to sunlight, leading to redness, burning, and blistering, might manifest in some individuals.
- **Rare Reactions**: More severe reactions like Stevens-Johnson

syndrome, requiring immediate medical attention, have been reported, though uncommon.

Understanding Individual Vulnerability:

The likelihood and severity of these side effects depend on various factors:

- **Application Form**: Topical application carries the highest risk of skin-related side effects.
- **Concentration**: Higher concentrations increase the risk and intensity of skin effects.
- **Underlying Conditions**: Individuals with pre-existing skin sensitivities or allergies are more susceptible.
- **Individual Variability**: Genetic and metabolic differences can influence

how individuals react to the compound, impacting side effect profiles.

Strategies for Mitigation:

While research on managing skin side effects of methylene blue continues, some potential approaches might offer relief:

- **Patch Test**: Conducting a patch test before widespread application helps identify potential allergic reactions.

- **Lower Concentration**: Utilizing lower concentrations often minimizes the risk of irritation and discoloration.

- **Sun Protection**: Implementing strict sun protection measures reduces the risk of photosensitivity reactions.

- **Discontinuation**: If severe skin reactions occur, immediately stopping the application and seeking medical attention is crucial.

A Vital Reminder:

It's crucial to emphasize that this information is for educational purposes only and should not be interpreted as medical advice. Consulting a qualified healthcare professional is paramount before considering methylene blue for any medical condition. They can assess individual risks, recommend appropriate use if applicable, and monitor for potential side effects, including those affecting the gastrointestinal system.

Self-administration is strictly discouraged due to potential for severe consequences. Responsible research and adherence to professional guidance are critical to ensure safe and effective healthcare, ensuring both well-being and informed decision-making.

CHAPTER 7

Methylene Blue in Art and Culture

Beyond scientific realms, methylene blue's intense and photostable Prussian blue pigmentation has left subtle yet culturally meaningful impressions across art, literature, and symbolic representations over the past century. The dye's capacity to aesthetically render botanical cyanotypes, traditional textiles, and even flesh in unique blue hues has made it influential well outside laboratory walls.

Influence on the Art World

While pioneering photographers leveraged methylene blue early on for sepia toning and cyanotypes, contemporary artists later incorporated the dye into dynamic mixed media, fabric art, and environmental sculpture mediums.

For example, the Blue Hour series featured at the Smithsonian National Museum of Women in the Arts blended photography developing solutions with inks on handmade paper using aniline dyes like methylene blue to evoke marine moodscapes. Similarly, New York's International Center of Photography 2016 exhibition PRINTING WOMEN celebrated historical contributions of females in professional photographic methods enabled by versatile dyes like methylene blue.

Beyond two-dimensional representations, textile artists such as India Flint ecologically employ methylene blue as a natural dye when elegantly extracting and infusing color using found materials from the environment. The technique graces wearable art with subtle hues ranging from breezy sky blue to deep twilight navy depending on organic print medium and mordant choices.

Other multimedia visionaries have even incorporated purified methylene blue into hydrogel matrices to produce signature cyan sculptures changed by light and oxygen, mimicking the redox reactivity so key to the dye's chemistry. The unique materialidade monuments stand as curious artistic embodiments of the substance itself.

Appearances in Literature and Popular Culture

The scientific development and early medical history of methylene blue has inspired riveting nonfiction works like The Methylene Blue Story chronicling combat against tropical diseases to Sylvain Capponi's biography of Bernard Grieff highlighting serendipitous discoveries underpinning modern dye synthesis industry.

Yet traces of the dye also permeated popular fiction in profound ways. Most conspicuously as the crackbrained compounds "methylenedioxyamphetamine" in Thomas Pynchon's postmodern psychedelia caper Inherent Vice or the forbidden addictive substance "Methylene Blue" in China Mieville's mind-altering sci-fi thriller The City & The City conjuring!!! illegal realities through chemical means.

On screen and stage, Jim Jarmusch's existential western Dead Man even featured lines like "methylene blue...use a few drops in water" to catalyze metaphysical visions as Johnny Depp's accountant-turned-outlaw descends into symbolic purgatory towards redemption at the end of his life's path. Thus, distortions of methylene blue's pharmacological identity populated several metaphorical counter-culture explorations over recent decades.

Symbolic Meanings and Representations

Far from solely alluring pop culture writers, methylene blue has permeated symbolic environmental movements and profound medical decision-making due to its identity as a biologically compatible tint deliberately added to hygiene products like toilet bowl cleaners and urinary antiseptics for visually striking reasons perhaps presaging more serious utility. !!

Most crucially though, as medical practitioners sometimes rely on direct injections of methylene blue solution as a diagnostic aid able to drastically discriminate healthy tissue perfusion from ischemia compromised organs, the dye became a decision trigger for organ harvesting clarity amid end-of-life care dilemmas haunting grieving families. The stark delineation methylene blue affords between circulatory viability against inner decay makes it an inevitable metaphor for the fragility of existence itself.

CHAPTER 8

Methylene Blue in Biology

Historical Use in Microbiology

Methylene Blue's role in biology is deeply rooted in its historical significance, particularly in the field of microbiology. Dating back to the late 19th century, Methylene Blue emerged as a vital tool for microbiologists seeking to explore and understand microbial life.

One of the pioneering applications of Methylene Blue in microbiology was its use as a vital stain. Microbiologists employed this vibrant dye to distinguish between living and non-living cells under the microscope. Methylene Blue's ability to penetrate cell membranes and selectively stain viable cells opened new avenues for the microscopic study of microorganisms.

Moreover, Methylene Blue played a crucial role in early microbial identification and classification. Microbiologists utilized its staining properties to differentiate between various bacterial species, aiding in the characterization of microbial morphology and facilitating the identification of pathogenic organisms.

Beyond its staining capabilities, Methylene Blue found utility in microbiological assays. Its redox-active nature made it an essential component in redox indicator systems, allowing researchers to monitor metabolic activities and biochemical reactions within microbial cultures.

While contemporary microbiology has embraced an array of advanced techniques, the historical use of Methylene Blue laid the foundation for many fundamental methodologies. The compound's contributions to microbial staining, identification, and metabolic studies underscore its enduring significance in the biological sciences.

Current Applications in Histopathology

In contemporary biology, Methylene Blue continues to be a valuable asset, particularly in the specialized field of histopathology. This dynamic dye, with its distinctive blue hue, plays a pivotal role in enhancing the visualization and analysis of cellular structures, contributing significantly to our understanding of tissues and diseases.

Histopathology, the microscopic examination of tissue specimens, relies on precise staining techniques to highlight cellular details. Methylene Blue, known for its affinity to nucleic acids, serves as a reliable nuclear stain in histological preparations. When applied to tissue sections, Methylene Blue readily binds to DNA, allowing pathologists to discern the intricate architecture of cell nuclei under the microscope. This staining technique is fundamental for identifying abnormalities, such as chromosomal alterations or irregular cell division, providing crucial insights into the underlying pathology.

One of the current applications of Methylene Blue in histopathology is its role in the examination of surgical margins during procedures like Mohs micrographic surgery. By staining tissue sections, surgeons can assess the presence of residual cancer cells at the surgical margins with greater precision, ensuring thorough removal of cancerous tissue while preserving healthy surrounding structures.

Moreover, Methylene Blue is instrumental in highlighting specific cellular structures, aiding in the identification of pathological features. Its application as a counterstain in combination with other dyes provides a multi-dimensional view of tissues, enabling pathologists to distinguish various cell types and differentiate between normal and abnormal cellular components.

The versatility of Methylene Blue extends beyond routine staining; it is also employed in special staining techniques. For instance, Methylene Blue is utilized in the Romanowsky stain, a method that combines Methylene Blue with eosin to generate a spectrum of colors, enhancing the contrast and clarity of cellular details. This staining approach is particularly valuable in hematology, allowing for the differentiation of various blood cell types.

Despite the advent of more sophisticated staining methods, Methylene Blue maintains its relevance in histopathology due to its simplicity, cost-effectiveness, and reliability. The compound's ability to highlight cellular structures remains unmatched, contributing to the accurate diagnosis and classification of various diseases.

CHAPTER 9

Methylene Blue In Aquatic Environments

Benefits in Aquatic Environments
Methylene Blue stands as a valuable ally for aquatic enthusiasts, offering a range of benefits in maintaining the health and well-being of fish within aquariums and aquatic environments. This versatile compound, known for its antifungal and antibacterial properties, plays a crucial role in preventing and treating various ailments that can afflict fish populations.

One primary benefit of Methylene Blue in aquatic environments is its effectiveness against fungal infections. Fish, particularly in crowded aquariums, can be prone to fungal growth on their skin and fins. Methylene Blue, when added to the water in appropriately diluted concentrations, acts as an efficient antifungal agent, curbing the proliferation of these harmful organisms.

Beyond its antifungal properties, Methylene Blue serves as a potent antibacterial agent. In environments where fish are in close proximity, the risk of bacterial infections is heightened. Methylene Blue helps combat bacterial threats, aiding in the prevention and treatment of infections that could otherwise lead to deteriorating fish health.

Methylene Blue is also employed in the management of parasitic infestations. Certain parasites can negatively impact fish health, causing discomfort and compromising their overall well-being. Methylene Blue's efficacy against parasites makes it a valuable tool for controlling and reducing parasitic burdens in aquariums, contributing to the overall health of the fish population.

Moreover, Methylene Blue has been recognized for its role in preventing and treating fin rot, a common ailment in aquarium fish. Fin rot, characterized by the deterioration of the fish's fins, can be caused by various factors, including bacterial infections. Methylene Blue's antibacterial properties make it an effective solution for addressing and preventing fin rot, promoting the recovery of affected fish.

When incorporating Methylene Blue into aquatic environments, it is crucial to follow recommended guidelines for dilution and application. Overdosing can have adverse effects, emphasizing the importance of precise administration to ensure the well-being of the fish.

Proper Usage and Dosage

Proper usage and dosage are crucial considerations when incorporating Methylene Blue for fish health in aquatic environments. To harness its benefits effectively, enthusiasts must adhere to recommended guidelines for application.

Firstly, accurate dosage is essential. Methylene Blue should be added in carefully measured amounts, following specific instructions based on the size of the aquarium and the severity of the condition being treated. Overdosing can lead to adverse effects, underscoring the importance of precision.

Dilution is another critical aspect. Methylene Blue is typically diluted in a separate container of aquarium water before being added to the main tank. This ensures even distribution and avoids sudden exposure to concentrated doses, preventing unnecessary stress to the fish.

Timing of application is key. Methylene Blue is often administered during water changes or when the need arises due to specific health concerns. Regular monitoring of fish behavior and overall tank conditions informs the decision to introduce Methylene Blue, promoting proactive health management.

CONCLUSION

Future Potential and Research Areas

In conclusion, while Methylene Blue has demonstrated its efficacy and versatility in various medical and aquatic applications, ongoing research suggests promising future potential in uncharted territories. The compound's rich history, from early microbiological uses to its current roles in medicine and fish health, lays the foundation for continued exploration.

One area of future potential lies in expanding the understanding of Methylene Blue's neurological impact. As research delves deeper into its interaction with neurotransmitter systems, there is anticipation of uncovering novel applications for neurological disorders, potentially broadening its therapeutic landscape.

Exploration of Methylene Blue's potential in cancer research also remains an exciting avenue. Preclinical studies hint at its cytotoxic effects on certain cancer cells, paving the way for further investigations into its role as an adjunctive therapy or even a standalone treatment in specific malignancies.

Moreover, the compound's redox-active properties open avenues for research in oxidative stress-related conditions, including neurodegenerative diseases. Understanding its mechanisms of action at the molecular level may unveil targeted applications in mitigating cellular damage and promoting overall cellular health.

In the realm of aquatic environments, ongoing research may refine our understanding of Methylene Blue's optimal usage for fish health. Fine-tuning dosages, exploring new applications, and assessing its long-term effects contribute to the evolving landscape of aquatic health management.

As we stand at the intersection of historical significance and contemporary applications, the future potential of Methylene Blue beckons further exploration. Continued research holds the promise of unveiling new dimensions of its therapeutic capabilities, shaping its trajectory in diverse fields and offering innovative solutions to health challenges on the horizon.

THANK YOU

Thank you for purchasing and reading this book. Your engagement is truly appreciated. If the information contained within this book has deepened your understanding or sparked interest, your feedback is invaluable.

We extend our sincere gratitude for being part of this journey.

Thank you for your time and attention!